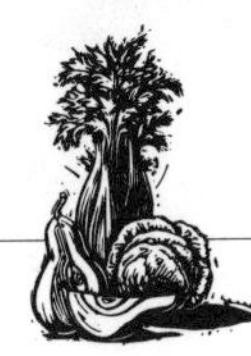

Contents

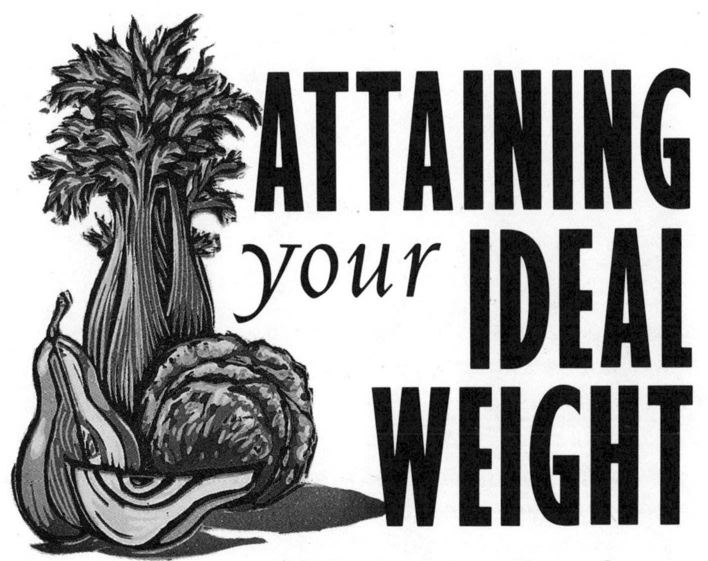

ATTAINING *your* IDEAL WEIGHT

With the Juice+Four Super-Nutrient Weight-Loss Plan

MICHAEL T. MURRAY, N.D.

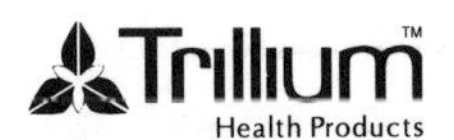

Seattle, Washington

Important

Please Read

The information in this book is intended to increase your knowledge of weight loss, nutrition and fresh fruit and vegetable juicing. By no means is it intended to diagnose or treat an individual's health problems or ailments. The information given is not medical advice nor is it presented as medical advice. Before starting any type of diet or weight-loss program, especially if you have more than 20 pounds to lose, please consult your own health care practitioner.

ISBN 0-9630948-2-3

Library of Congress Catalog Card Number: 92-61628

Cover illustrations by Kris Wiltse.

Printed in the United States of America.

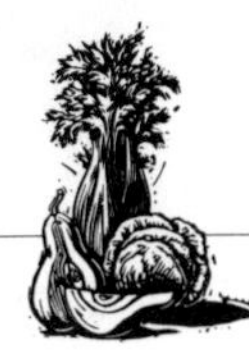

Introduction

Why do some people gain weight so easily, while others eat all they want and never seem to put on a pound? And why do so many people find it extremely difficult to lose weight, while others have difficulty keeping weight on? What is the best approach for permanent results? What is the best diet? Researchers have sought answers to these questions for decades, but we're still plagued by many myths and misconceptions about obesity. Many individuals, including some physicians, falsely believe that obesity is just a matter of poor eating habits or lack of proper nutrition education. In addition, in recent years, the psychological aspects of obesity have been overstated. The psychological understanding of obesity ties overeating directly to external cues, such as sight, smell and taste. The result is a tremendous stigma felt by many individuals who are overweight.

However, more and more research is supporting a biological basis for obesity. In other words, the signals telling us whether or not to eat appear to be internal—tied directly to the biochemical activity of the fat cells themselves. This approach offers renewed hope for individuals who have tried diets, behavioral modification and many other weight-loss methods without much success. Understanding obesity in terms of the way in which our bodies react to the food we eat is leading to more effective methods for not only losing weight, but even more importantly, keeping the weight off.

It is clear that both the biological and the psychological needs of the individual must be addressed. Any successful, healthy, weight-loss and weight-maintenance plan should incorporate effective strategies for developing a positive mental attitude, a regular and appropriate exercise program, and most importantly, consistent healthy food choices that provide the body with high quality nutrition. This book addresses each of these important issues and introduces Juice+Four—the super-nutrient meal replacement developed by Trillium Health Products to meet the nutritional demands of your body and help you attain your ideal weight for optimum health.

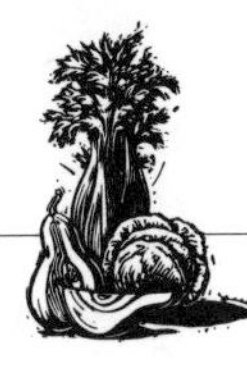

1
What is Obesity?

The simplest definition of *obesity* is an excessive amount of body fat. This must be distinguished from the term *overweight*, which refers to an excess of body weight relative to height. For example, a muscular athlete may be overweight, yet have a very low body fat percentage. What causes him or her to be overweight is muscle or lean body mass, not excess body fat. Despite the fact that weight alone does not always reflect an accurate body fat percentage, obesity is often defined as a weight greater than 20 percent more than the average desirable weight for men and women of a given height.

Many physicians and nutritionists get more precise estimates of body fat percentage with methods such as skinfold thickness, bioelectric impedance and ultrasound. When these more accurate techniques are used, obesity is better defined as a body fat percentage greater than 30 percent for women and greater than 25 percent for men.[1,2]

The most popular height and weight charts are the tables of

"desirable weight" provided by the Metropolitan Life Insurance Company. The most recent edition of these tables, published in 1983, gives weight ranges for men and women at one inch increments of height for three body frame sizes. Many nutrition experts, however, have been reluctant to use the 1983 table due to its higher weight range compared to earlier tables. The 1983 Metropolitan Height and Weight tables are provided opposite.

To make a simple determination of your frame size, extend your arm and bend the forearm upwards at a 90 degree angle. Keep your fingers straight and turn the inside of your wrist away from your body. Place the thumb and index finger of your other hand on the two prominent bones on either side of your elbow. Carefully measure the space between your fingers. Compare that measurement with the following figures given for medium-framed individuals. A reading lower than that on the chart indicates a small frame; a higher reading indicates a large frame.

Determining Frame Size

Women—Medium Frame		**Men—Medium Frame**	
Height in 1" heels	*Elbow breadth*	*Height in 1" heels*	*Elbow breadth*
4'10" – 5'3"	2 1/4" – 2 1/2"	5'2" – 5'3"	2 1/2" – 2 7/8"
5'4" – 5'11"	2 3/8" – 2 5/8"	5'4" – 5'7"	2 5/8" – 2 7/8"
6'0"	2 1/2" – 2 3/4"	5'8" – 5'11"	2 3/4" – 3"
		6'0" – 6'3"	2 3/4" – 3 1/8"
		6'4"	2 7/8" – 3 1/4"

Classification and Types of Obesity

Obesity is often classified into three major categories based on the size and number of fat (adipose) cells. Fat cells may be increased in number, which is called hyperplastic obesity; fat cells may be increased in size, which is called hypertrophic obesity; or fat cells may be increased in both number and size, which is called hyperplastic-hypertrophic obesity.

1983 Metropolitan Height and Weight Table

Weights for adults age 25 to 59 years based on lowest mortality. Weight in pounds according to frame size in indoor clothing (5 pounds for men and 3 pounds for women) wearing shoes with 1-inch heels.

	Small Frame	*Medium Frame*	*Large Frame*
Women			
4'10"	102-111	109-121	118-131
4'11"	103-113	111-123	120-134
5'0"	104-115	113-126	122-137
5'1"	106-118	115-129	125-140
5'2"	108-121	118-132	128-143
5'3"	111-124	121-135	131-147
5'4"	114-127	124-138	134-151
5'5"	117-130	127-141	137-155
5'6"	120-133	130-144	140-159
5'7"	123-136	133-147	143-163
5'8"	126-139	136-150	146-167
5'9"	129-142	139-153	149-170
5'10"	132-145	142-156	152-173
5'11"	135-148	145-159	155-176
6'0"	138-151	148-162	158-179
Men			
5'2"	128-134	131-141	138-150
5'3"	130-136	133-143	140-153
5'4"	132-138	135-145	142-156
5'5"	134-140	137-148	144-160
5'6"	136-142	139-151	146-164
5'7"	138-145	142-154	149-168
5'8"	140-148	145-157	152-172
5'9"	142-151	148-160	155-176
5'10"	144-154	151-163	158-180
5'11"	146-157	154-166	161-184
6'0"	149-160	157-170	164-188
6'1"	152-164	160-174	168-192
6'2"	155-168	164-178	172-197
6'3"	158-172	167-182	176-202
6'4"	162-176	171-187	181-207

The development of too many fat cells (hyperplastic obesity) usually begins in childhood. Although it predisposes an individual to a life-long battle with his or her weight, interestingly, this form of obesity tends to be associated with fewer health risks than hypertrophic obesity. Hypertrophic obesity, an increase in the size of fat cells, usually develops later on in life and is generally associated with weight gain in the torso. Hypertrophic obesity is associated more with the metabolic complications of obesity, such as diabetes, high blood pressure, and high cholesterol and triglyceride levels. When there is both an increased number and increased size of fat cells, it is extremely difficult to achieve ideal body weight.

Male-patterned (android) and female-patterned (gynecoid) obesity refer to classifications of obesity based on fat distribution. In android obesity, fat is deposited primarily in the upper body and abdomen. This type of obesity is typically seen in the obese male, hence the term male-patterned or android obesity. A waist girth greater than the hip girth is considered an indicator of android obesity.[3,4]

In female-patterned or gynecoid obesity, the fat is distributed primarily in the lower body in the buttocks and thighs. This obesity pattern is most typically observed in females, hence the term female-patterned or gynecoid obesity.[3,4]

In general, android obesity is associated with more serious metabolic disorders, especially diabetes. In addition to this link to diabetes, android obesity, whether in men or women, has been shown to significantly increase the risk for heart disease. Android obesity is often associated with high blood pressure and high cholesterol levels, as well as gallstones and endocrine diseases.[5-8]

Psychological Aspects

The current psychological view of obesity assumes that excessive eating is due to psychological or emotional reasons. The main belief of the psychological approach is that obese individuals eat in response to external cues and stimuli (sight, smell and taste), even when their appetite is satisfied.[1,2] For example, television watching has been linked very strongly with obesity. Studies have shown that the number of hours spent watching television is the strongest predictor for becoming obese.[9] The more TV watched, the greater the likelihood and degree of obesity. This fits in very well with the psychological theory (increased sensitivity to external cues), as watching TV has also been shown to result in increased food consumption.

However, watching TV has several biological effects that promote obesity. A significant reduction in physical activity is associated with watching television, and a lowering of the metabolic rate to a level similar to that experienced during trance-like states. These factors can clearly affect the body's metabolism and contribute to obesity as much as excessive eating habits.[1,10]

Psychological therapy is designed to replace food consumption stimuli with new cues to reduce food intake. Unfortunately, when used alone, this approach has not been very successful.[11] This could be because obese individuals can still put on weight even when consuming far fewer calories than their lean counterparts. This indicates that the biological factors involved also play a very important role in obesity. That is, it is not simply the amount of food that is eaten, but also the types of food and the way the body and fat cells react to our eating habits that cause obesity.

Another important psychological factor to be considered is the stigma attached to being obese. A group of children were once asked if they would rather be fat or physically disabled. The results of the study were clear: children would rather be physically disabled than fat. Obese individuals experience much psychological trauma to their self-esteem. Fashion trends, insurance programs, college placements, employment opportunities—all can discriminate against the obese person. Consequently, the obese person learns many self-defeating and self-degrading attitudes. They are led to believe that fat is "bad," which often results in a vicious cycle of low self-esteem, depression, overeating for consolation, increased obesity, social rejection and further lowering of self-esteem. Counseling is often necessary to change attitudes about being obese and to aid in the improvement of self-esteem. If self-esteem is not considered, even the most perfect diet and exercise plan will fail. Improving the way overweight people feel about themselves assists them in changing their eating behaviors.

Biological Aspects

While the psychological theory proposes that obese individuals don't respond to internal feelings of hunger and satiety, the biological theory states almost the opposite: obese individuals appear to be extremely sensitive to these internal clues.[12] The biological or biochemical models of obesity are tied to the metabolism of the fat cells. These models support the notion that obesity is not just a matter of overeating, and explain why some people can eat very large quantities of calories and not increase their weight substantially, while for the obese just the reverse is true.

Research with animals and humans has found that each individual has a "set point" or target weight programmed into the fat cells, which the body tries to maintain. One theory is that the fat cells themselves control this set point; when the fat cell becomes smaller (such as any time there is a lack of food), it sends a message to the brain to eat. Since the obese individual often has both more and larger fat cells, and because these cells seem to be more sensitive to fluctuation in size, the result is an overpowering urge to eat.

This explains why most diets don't work. While the obese individual can fight off the impulse for a time, eventually the signal becomes too strong to ignore. The result is rebound overeating with individuals often exceeding their previous weight. In addition, their set point, the weight which the body strives to maintain, is now set at a higher level—the fat cells have increased in size and think they need to stay this way—making it even more difficult to lose weight.[13] This is known as the "yo-yo" or "ratchet" effect.

The set point seems to be tied to the sensitivity of fat cells to insulin. Insulin is a hormone secreted by the pancreas. Its primary function is to help regulate blood sugar levels by promoting the absorption of blood glucose by cells of the body. Normally, when sufficient blood glucose has been absorbed for the body's current energy needs, the feeling of hunger diminishes. However, if blood sugar or glucose is absorbed more rapidly than it can be used by the body for energy, it is stored as fat. Obesity leads to insulin insensitivity and vice versa. When cells become insensitive to insulin, blood sugar levels reach higher than normal levels. This is known as diabetes. Both obesity and diabetes are strongly linked to the so-called "Western diet," presumably due to the harmful effects refined sugar has on insulin and blood sugar control mechanisms.[14]

The key to overcoming the fat cells' set point appears to be increasing the sensitivity of the fat cells to insulin. The set point theory suggests that a weight-loss plan that does not improve insulin sensitivity will most likely fail to provide long-term results. Insulin sensitivity can be improved, and the set point lowered, by exercise and a specially designed program that provides greater nutrition through healthy food choices.

The Weight-Loss Equation

Weight loss is perhaps one of the most challenging health goals. Few people want to be overweight, yet only 5 percent of markedly obese individuals, and only 66 percent of people just a few pounds or so overweight, are able to achieve and maintain "normal" body weight.[1,2,10]

Literally hundreds of diets and diet programs claim to provide the answer to the problem of obesity. Dieters are constantly bombarded with new reports of "wonder" diets to follow. However, the basic equation for losing weight never changes. In order for an individual to lose weight, calorie intake must be less than the amount of calories burned. This can only be accomplished by decreasing food intake and/or increasing physical activity.

To lose one pound of fat, a person must take in 3,500 fewer calories than he or she expends. To lose three pounds of fat each week, there must be a negative caloric balance of 1,000 calories a day. To reduce one's caloric intake by 1,000 calories is often difficult, as is burning an additional 1,000 calories per day by exercise (a person would need to jog for 90 minutes, play tennis for 2 hours, or take a brisk two and one half hour walk). The most sensible approach to weight loss is to decrease caloric intake and exercise simultaneously.

Successful permanent weight loss must incorporate high quality nutrition, regular physical exercise and psychological support for a positive mental attitude. All these components are critical and interrelated; no single component is more important than another. Improvement in one area may result in some positive changes, but improving all three yields the greatest results.

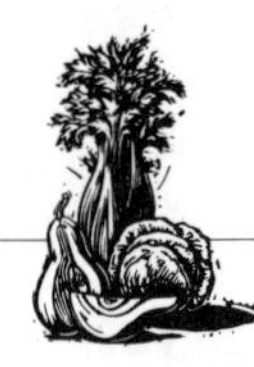

2
Psychological Support

Increasing self-esteem and promoting a healthy positive mental attitude are critical factors in a successful weight-loss program. In order to achieve these goals, you need to exercise or condition your mind just as you condition your body. The following exercises are designed to help you achieve the kind of permanent results you really want by conditioning you for success. You will need to get a notebook that you can write in. This will become your personal journal. A journal is a powerful tool to help you stay in touch with your feelings, thoughts and emotions. The exercises that follow are designed to help you learn how to adopt healthier attitudes. These exercises will provide the foundation for a positive mental outlook. Your daily personal journal will build upon this foundation. If you do not have a notebook you can use as a journal, and you want to begin right now, find some paper that you can write on and enter your answers to the following questions.

Exercise #1

Creating Your Positive Goal Statement

Learning to set goals in a way that results in a positive experience is critical to your success. The following guidelines can be used to set any goal, including attaining your desired weight. You can use goal setting to create a "success cycle." Achieving goals helps you feel better about yourself, and the better you feel about yourself, the more likely you will achieve your goals.

State the goal in positive terms. Do not use any negative words in your goal statement. For example, it is better to say "I enjoy eating healthy, low-calorie, nutritious foods" than "I will not eat sugar, candy, ice cream and other fattening foods." Remember, always state the goal in positive terms and do not use any negative words in the goal statement.

Make your goal attainable and realistic. For example, if you are just beginning a walking program, set your goal at a short distance that you know you can achieve. You will then have the confidence to increase your distance goals gradually over time. Again, goals can be used to create a success cycle and positive self image. Little things add up to make a major difference in the way you feel about yourself.

Be specific. The more clearly your goal is defined, the more likely you are to reach it. What is the weight you desire? What is the body fat percentage or measurements you desire? Clearly define what it is you want to achieve.

State the goal in the present tense, not the future tense. In order to reach your goal, you have to believe you have already attained it. As noted psychologist Dr. Wayne Dyer says "You'll see it, when you believe it." You must literally program yourself to achieve your goal. See and feel yourself having already achieved the goal and success will be yours. Remember, always state your goal in the present tense.

✍ **Use the guidelines above to construct a positive goal statement.**

For example: "*My body is strong and beautiful. I have a 23 percent body fat percentage and I weigh 125 pounds. I feel good about myself and my body. I am losing 2 pounds a week with the help of my new weight-loss plan and I feel fantastic!*"

Any voyage begins with one step and is followed by many other steps. Short-term goals can be used to help you achieve those long-term results described in your positive goal statement. Get in the habit of asking yourself the following question each morning and evening: What must I do today to achieve my long term goal?

Exercise #2

Are You Ready to Lose Weight Now?

Now that you have created your positive goal statement, how committed are you to achieving your goal? Without commitment, there can be no success. If you can absolutely commit to achieving your goal, nothing can stand in your way. By reading the following passage to yourself, you will be stating that you are committed to reaching your desired weight *right now*.

> "Until one is committed there is hesitancy, the chance to draw back, always ineffectiveness. Concerning all acts of initiative (and creation), there is one elementary truth, the ignorance of which kills countless ideas and splendid plans: that the moment one definitely commits oneself, then Providence moves too. All sorts of things occur to help one that would never have otherwise occurred. A whole stream of events issues from the decision raising in one's favor all manner of unforeseen incidents and meetings and material assistance which no man could have dreamed would have come his way. Whatever you can do, or dream you can, begin it. Boldness has genius, power and magic in it. Begin it now!" ~GOETHE

✍ **To reinforce this commitment, write out the answers to the following questions:**

- What is the pleasure you have gotten by not losing weight?
- What is the pain that has kept you from losing weight?
- What pain would you experience in the future if you didn't lose weight?
- What will you have to gain by losing weight?
- Give ten reasons why you absolutely must lose weight right now.
- Give ten reasons why you absolutely can lose weight right now.

Exercise #3

The Power of Questions

According to Anthony Robbins, author of the best sellers *Unlimited Power* and *Awakening the Giant Within,* the quality of your life is equal to the quality of the questions you habitually ask yourself. This is based on the belief that whatever question you ask your brain—you will get an answer.

Let's look at the following example: An individual is met with a particular challenge or problem. He or she can ask a number of questions when in this situation. One question many people ask in this circumstance is "Why does this always happen to me?" Do they get an answer? Do the answers build self-esteem? Does the problem keep reappearing? What would be a higher quality question? How about, "This is a very interesting situation—what do I need to learn from this situation?" Or, "What can I do to make this situation better?" If you want to have a better life, simply ask better questions. It sounds simple, because it is.

✍ **To help you achieve not only your desired weight, but also a happier life, ask yourself the following questions on a consistent basis, and write out your answers in your journal.**

Morning Questions

- What am I most happy about in my life right now?
  Why does that make me happy?
  How does that make me feel?
- What am I most excited about in my life right now?
  Why does that make me excited?
  How does that make me feel?
- What am I most grateful about in my life right now?
  Why does that make me grateful?
  How does that make me feel?
- What am I enjoying most about in my life right now?
  What about that do I enjoy?
  How does that make me feel?
- What am I committed to in my life right now?
  Why am I committed to that?
  How does that make me feel?
- Who do I love? (Starting close, and moving out.)
  Who loves me?
- What must I do today to achieve my long-term goal?

Evening Questions

- What have I given today?
  In what ways have I been a giver today?
- What did I learn today?
- In what ways was today a perfect day?
- Repeat morning questions.

Problem or Challenge Questions

- What is right/great about this problem or challenge?
- What is not perfect yet?
- What am I willing to do to make it the way I want?
- How can I enjoy doing the things necessary to make it the way I want it?

Exercise #4

Affirmations

An affirmation is a positive statement. Affirmations can make imprints on the subconscious mind to create a healthy, positive self image. In addition, affirmations can actually fuel the changes you desire. The following are guidelines for effective affirmations:

Choose a location that is comfortable and quiet, and a time when you will not be interrupted or disturbed.

Sit or lie in a comfortable position. Relax by breathing deeply and slowly. Inhale to a count of one, hold for a count of two, and exhale to a count of four.

Always phrase an affirmation in the present tense.

Always phrase the affirmation in a positive way and totally associate with the positive feelings that are generated.

Keep the affirmation short and simple, but full of feeling.

Be creative. Imagine yourself really experiencing what you are affirming.

Make the affirmation personal and full of meaning.

The following are some examples of positive affirmations:

- I am a whole and complete person. I am in control of my life.
- I am an open channel of love and joy.
- I am filled with peace and wisdom.
- I am good to my body.
- I am growing stronger every day.
- I am healthier and thinner every day.

✍ **Using the above guidelines and examples, write down five affirmations regarding eating healthfully. State these affirmations aloud for a total of five minutes each day.**

✍ **Now write down five affirmations about physical activity. State these affirmations aloud for a total of five minutes each day.**

Your Personal Journal

Your personal journal will serve as a testimony to your success. In your journal, keep a checklist to make sure you have performed all of the daily exercises. Also enter a daily diet summary.

✍ **Maintain a checklist of the following daily exercises:**

___ Morning Questions
___ Weight Check
___ Goal Statement
___ Evening Questions
___ Affirmations

✍ **Enter a daily diet summary:**

- Breakfast
- Lunch
- Snacks
- Dinner

✍ **Other daily diary entries:**

- Physical activity
- Little things that made this day special
- The most successful triumph of the day
- Other comments

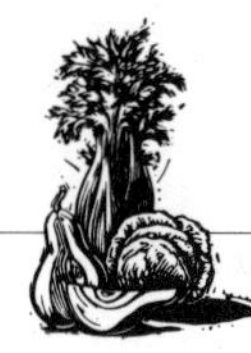

3
Physical Exercise

The health benefits of regular exercise cannot be overstated. The immediate effect of exercise is stress on the body; however, with a regular exercise program, the body adapts. The body's response to this regular stress is that it becomes stronger, functions more efficiently, and has greater endurance. Exercise is a vital component in a successful, permanent weight-loss plan.[15]

Physical inactivity may be a major cause of obesity in the U.S. Indeed, childhood obesity seems to be associated more with inactivity than overeating, and strong evidence suggests that 80 to 86 percent of adult obesity begins in childhood. In the adult population, obese adults are less active than their leaner counterparts.[16] Regular exercise is a necessary component of a successful weight-loss program due to the following factors:

1. When weight loss is achieved by dieting without exercise, a substantial portion of the total weight loss comes from the lean tissue, primarily as water loss.[17]

2. When exercise is included in a weight-loss program, overall body composition usually improves due to a gain in lean body weight because of an increase in muscle mass and a corresponding decrease in body fat.[18]
3. Exercise helps counter the reduction in basal metabolic rate (BMR) that usually accompanies calorie restriction alone.[19]
4. Exercise increases the BMR for an extended period of time following the exercise session.[20]
5. Moderate to intense exercise may have an appetite suppressant effect.[20]
6. Those individuals who exercise during and after weight reduction are better able to maintain their weight loss than those who do not exercise.[21]

Physical Benefits

The entire body benefits from regular exercise, largely as a result of improved cardiovascular and respiratory function. Simply stated, exercise enhances the transport of oxygen and nutrients into cells. At the same time, exercise enhances the transport of carbon dioxide and waste products from the tissues of the body to the blood stream and ultimately to the eliminative organs.

Regular exercise is particularly important in reducing the risk of heart disease. It does this by lowering cholesterol levels, improving blood and oxygen supply to the heart, increasing the functional capacity of the heart, reducing blood pressure, reducing obesity, and exerting a favorable effect on blood clotting.

Psychological and Social Benefits

Regular exercise makes people not only look better, but also makes them feel better. Tensions, depressions, feelings of inadequacy and worries diminish greatly with regular exercise. The value of an exercise program in the treatment of depression cannot be overstated. Exercise alone has been demonstrated to have a tremendous impact on improving mood and the ability to handle stressful life situations. A recent study published in the American Journal of Epidemiology shows that increased participation in exercise, sports and physical activities is strongly associated with decreased symptoms of:

- Depression (feelings that life is not worthwhile, low spirits)
- Anxiety (restlessness, tension)
- Malaise (feeling run down, insomnia)[22]

How to Start

The first thing to do is make sure you are fit enough to start an exercise program. If you have been mostly inactive for a number of years, or have any medical condition that could be aggravated by exercise, such as heart problems, diabetes, high cholesterol, arthritis, recent injury or surgery, or being more than 30 pounds overweight, see your physician first. You may need the help of a professional in designing a personalized exercise program.

If you are fit enough to begin, the next thing to do is select an activity you feel you would enjoy. The best exercises are the kind that get your heart moving. Aerobic activities such as walking briskly, jogging, bicycling, cross-country skiing, swimming, aerobic dance and racquet sports are good examples. Brisk walking (5 miles an hour) for approximately 30 minutes may be the very best form of exercise for weight loss. Walking can be done anywhere, it doesn't require any expensive equipment (just comfortable clothing and well-fitting shoes) and the risk for injury is extremely low.

The concept of "spot reduction" is a myth.[23] Exercise draws from all of the fat stores of the body, not just from local deposits. While aerobic exercise generally enhances weight-loss programs, weight-training programs can also substantially alter body composition by increasing lean body weight and decreasing body fat.[24,25]

Thus, weight training may be just as, or more, effective than aerobic exercise in maintaining or increasing lean body weight and, therefore, the metabolic rate of individuals undergoing weight reduction.

Intensity of Exercise

Exercise intensity is determined by measuring your heart rate, the number of times your heart beats per minute. This can be quickly done by placing your index and middle finger of one hand on the side of the neck just below the angle of the jaw, or on the opposite wrist. Beginning with zero, count the number of pulses for 6 seconds. Simply add a zero to this number and you have your pulse. For example, if you counted 14 beats, your heart rate would be 140. Would this be a good number? It depends upon your training zone.

A quick and easy way to determine your maximum training heart rate is to subtract your age from 185. For example, if you are 40 years old your maximum heart rate would be 145. To determine the bottom of the training zone, simply subtract 20 from your maximum heart rate. In the case of a 40-year-old, this would be 125. So, the training range would be between 125 and 145 beats per minute. For maximum health benefits, you must stay in this range and never exceed it.

Duration and Frequency

A minimum of 15 to 20 minutes of exercise at your training heart rate at least three times a week is necessary to gain any significant benefits from exercise. It is better to exercise at the lower end of your training zone for longer periods of time than it is to exercise at a higher intensity for shorter periods of time. It is also better if you can make exercise a part of your daily routine.

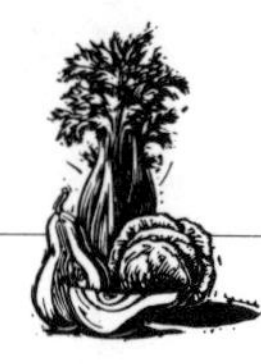

4
Healthy Food Choices

Healthy food choices comprise the third, and perhaps most important, element of effective weight loss. As previously mentioned, it is not simply the amount of food that is eaten but also the type of food that is critical for permanent, healthy weight loss. A properly balanced, nutrient packed diet will not only help support your health during weight loss, it will help curb feelings of hunger. Food choices are also very important to your general health: over one-half of all chronic degenerative diseases (such as heart attack, lung disease, stroke and arthritis) are diet related, and can be prevented and in some cases even treated through longstanding dietary modifications.

More and more nutrition authorities are recommending a vegetarian or nearly-vegetarian diet. One group, the Physicians Committee for Responsible Medicine, has proposed the New Four Food Groups. This plan eliminates animal products altogether in its four categories: whole grains, vegetables, legumes and fruits. The New Four Food Groups is not only healthier in its reliance on foods lower on the food chain, it is also a more environmentally sensitive eating plan.

Because both weight loss and our general health are so closely linked to proper nutrition, the Juice+Four plan offers a nutritional supplement of superior content and effectiveness, and emphasizes a diet based on the New Four Food Groups.

Juice+Four

To help people attain their ideal weight, and to help them keep the nutrient levels of their diets high, Trillium Health Products has developed the Juice+Four Meal Replacement Formula. Juice+Four, along with fresh juice and the dietary recommendations made further in this chapter, is designed to provide approximately 1,200 to 1,500 calories per day. This, along with aerobic exercise for 15 to 20 minutes, three to four times per week, will produce optimum weight loss at a rate of approximately 1 to 3 pounds per week. Starvation and crash diets usually result in rapid weight loss (largely muscle and water), but cause rebound weight gain (remember the set point?). The most successful approach to weight loss is gradual weight reduction through adopting longstanding dietary and lifestyle modifications. This is the goal of the Juice+Four Plan.

This formula represents a major breakthrough in meal replacement formulas. Juice+Four is designed to mix with fresh fruit and vegetable juices and to provide a healthy balance of the New Four Food Groups. Juice+Four is a natural vegetarian formula providing the following benefits:

- High quality protein from grains and legumes
- A rich source of soluble and insoluble dietary fibers
- Balanced, high-quality nutrition with enhanced levels of nutrients critical during weight loss
- Low total fat content, but a rich source of important essential fatty acids
- No sweeteners, artificial flavors, or other artificial foods

Protein Quality

The protein quality of Juice+Four is extremely high. To determine the quality, a method known as the "protein efficiency ratio" or PER is used. This is calculated based on a protein source's ability to promote growth in young animals. Casein, a milk protein, is often used as the standard of comparison. By balancing the ratio of grains to legumes, the PER of Juice+Four is 2.5, the same as casein. However, the mixture of protein sources in Juice+Four is far superior to casein.

Casein is often difficult for people to digest and many people are allergic to it. Casein is used not only in many meal replacement formulas, it is also used in glues, molded plastics and paints. More and more concerned people are avoiding casein and are instead looking for vegetarian alternatives. Juice+Four provides an excellent mixture of soy, pea, wheat and rice protein.

Each serving of Juice+Four provides 15 grams of high quality protein. The major protein component of Juice+Four is Supro,™ the only soy protein blend with extensive research behind it. Supro meets, or exceeds, all essential amino acid requirements as set by the World Health Organization.[29] In addition, extensive research has demonstrated not only Supro's high protein efficiency ratio (PER), high digestibility and low allergic nature, but that Supro is well-tolerated and promotes weight loss, lowers cholesterol levels, and improves blood sugar control.[29-35]

The vegetarian protein mixture in Juice+Four provides significant advantages over other commonly used protein sources for meal replacement formulas. For example, experimental studies in animals and humans have shown that vegetarian protein sources, such as soy protein, tend to lower cholesterol levels while protein from animal sources, particularly casein from milk, tend to raise cholesterol levels.[35-38] A great deal of research has been dedicated to find out if this effect is due to the protein components or some other component in the foods.

Although the nonprotein components of vegetarian protein

supplement products may have a mild cholesterol-lowering effect, the major cholesterol-lowering action is due to the protein components.[36] Researchers have yet to determine exactly how vegetable protein lowers cholesterol levels, as several factors have been observed which would account for the reduction. The cholesterol-lowering effect of soy protein formulations are more apparent when serum cholesterol levels are high. Studies have shown that total and LDL cholesterol are both reduced, as are elevated triglyceride levels.[36]

From a practical perspective, consumers should be wary of casein containing (i.e.,milk-based) meal replacement formulas. Casein has been shown to not only increase cholesterol levels, but increase the development of gallstones as well.[35-38] In contrast, soy-based meal replacement formulas like Juice+Four actually lower cholesterol levels.[36]

Fiber Blend Benefits

Juice+Four provides both soluble and insoluble fibers from oat fiber, soy polysaccharide (Fibrim™), rice fiber, citrus pectin, apple fiber, beet fiber, guar gum, gum arabic, corn bran and purified cellulose. Each serving provides a total of 6 grams of fiber with 65 percent being insoluble fiber and 35 percent being soluble fiber. Insoluble fibers, like oat fiber, Fibrim, beet fiber, corn bran and cellulose promote proper bowel function, while soluble fiber exerts a number of important actions useful in promoting weight loss. Soluble fibers, like pectin, guar gum and gum arabic, slow down the absorption of sugar into the bloodstream, thereby leading to improved carbohydrate metabolism. They also reduce appetite.[1,2]

The fibers contained in Juice+Four:

- Promote improved bowel function
- Delay gastric emptying, resulting in reduced elevations of blood glucose levels after a meal
- Increase feelings of fullness
- Decrease appetite
- Increase pancreatic secretions

- Increase stool weight
- Promote more advantageous intestinal microflora
- Increase production of short chain fatty acids
- Decrease serum cholesterol and lipids
- Produce a more soluble bile

It is well established that a fiber-deficient diet is an important factor in the development of obesity.[14] Dietary fiber plays a role in preventing obesity by:

- Slowing the eating process
- Increasing fecal caloric loss
- Altering digestive hormone secretion
- Improving glucose tolerance
- Inducing satiety by increased gastric filling, stimulation of the release of appetite suppressing hormones like cholecysto-kinin, and intestinal bulking action.

Perhaps the prime effects of fiber on obesity are related to improving glucose metabolism. Blood sugar disorders (hypoglycemia and diabetes) appear to be most clearly related to inadequate dietary fiber intake.[14] Clinical trials have demonstrated the beneficial effects of several water soluble fibers (such as guar gum, gum karaya and pectin) on blood sugar control.[1,2,39]

In the treatment of obesity, dietary fiber supplementation has been shown to promote weight loss. Its main action appears to be reducing caloric consumption by increasing the feeling of fullness and decreasing the feeling of hunger.[39-42] Juice+Four provides an ideal mixture of fiber sources that mix easily in fresh juice.

Enhanced Nutrition

Juice+Four provides key nutrients necessary during weight loss. In addition to the high quality protein and fiber complexes in Juice+Four, 27 vitamins and minerals are provided, including high levels of absorbable calcium. Juice+Four is especially rich in trace elements like chromium, selenium, molybdenum, manganese and vanadium. The Standard American Diet (SAD) is often lacking in these nutrients, a factor which may contribute to obesity. For example, the trace mineral chromium functions in the "glucose tolerance factor," a critical enzyme system in blood sugar regulation.[1,43-45] In fact, considerable evidence now indicates that chromium levels are a major determinant of insulin sensitivity. Remember that one of the theories explaining why so many Americans are obese is a decreased sensitivity to insulin. Chromium deficiency may be a contributing factor.

Reversing a chromium deficiency by supplementing the diet with chromium has been demonstrated to lower body weight yet increase lean body mass, improve glucose tolerance, and decrease total cholesterol and triglyceride levels.[1,43,44] All these effects appear due to increased insulin sensitivity. In Juice+Four, chromium is supplied by ChromeMate GTF™ (chromium polynicotinate), an extensively researched and well accepted source of highly absorbable chromium.[45] The trace minerals manganese and vanadium are also important co-factors in key enzymes of sugar metabolism.[1]

Essential Fatty Acids

The Juice+Four Meal Replacement Formula is low in calories from fat; only 8 percent of the calories are provided from fats. However, the fat provided by Juice+Four is essential because it is provided by essential fatty acids. These oils are termed "essential" because our bodies cannot manufacture them. They function as components in our cell membranes and in the manufacture of biological compounds.

The source of the essential fatty acids in Juice+Four is canola oil. This oil was chosen because it provides a rich source of polyunsaturated fatty acids in a good ratio. Canola oil provides both omega-6 essential fatty acids (like linoleic acid) and omega-3 fatty acids (like alpha-linolenic acid). Soy lecithin is included in the formula because it facilitates the absorption of the essential fatty acids and is itself a rich source of essential fatty acids.

What is Not in Juice+Four

It's not only what is in Juice+Four that makes it the most ideal meal replacement formula, it is also what is not in it. Most meal replacement formulas are full of sugar, artificial colors and flavors, aspartame (NutraSweet™), and other food additives. Most people are aware of the negative effects of too much sugar in our diets. Refined sugar leads to loss of blood sugar control, diabetes and obesity.[14] Sucrose (white table sugar), fructose, or corn syrup are the first ingredients of many meal replacement formulas. Obviously, these should be avoided if permanent weight loss is desired. In contrast, Juice+Four contains no added sugar or food additives.

More and more food additives, like preservatives, artificial colors, artificial flavorings and acidifiers, are being shown to be extremely detrimental to our health. In fact, many food additives have been banned due to their cancer causing effects, and many other synthetic food additives are currently being linked to a wide variety of diseases. Meal replacement formulas containing artificial food additives should be avoided.

The Basic Juice+Four Plan

During the first week of the Juice+Four Super-Nutrient Weight-Loss Plan, three daily Juice+Four meals are recommended. Each of these meals consists of one serving of Juice+Four mixed with 12 ounces of fresh juice. During this week your body will begin ridding itself of stored toxins. Substances toxic to our bodies are everywhere. In the air we breathe, the food we eat and the water we drink. Even our bodies and the bacteria in our intestines produce toxic substances. The health of an individual is largely determined by the ability of the body to "detoxify." Juice+Four, along with fresh juice, provides key nutrients which will help your body deal with and eliminate these harmful substances. As you continue on the program, your body will continue to eliminate these stored toxins. Your body needs the protection of fresh juice, Juice+Four and a high-fiber diet.

After week 1, and until your target weight is reached, we recommend two Juice+Four meals plus a third meal of wholesome foods from the New Four Food Groups (grains, legumes, fruits and vegetables). This plant-based diet will provide your body with important fiber and nutrients. It will also provide continued support for enhanced detoxification.

The harmful effects of "yo-yoing" weight are clear. That is why Juice+Four is also designed for weight maintenance. If you see one or two pounds creeping back on, substitute one or more daily solid meals with Juice+Four mixed with your favorite juice. It is also recommended that you increase your physical activity until you are back at your target weight. Juice+Four is also ideal as a daily nutritional supplement. Remember, by substituting one Juice+Four meal for one solid meal, you're getting one-third of your daily RDA in a quick, low-calorie "meal-in-a-glass."

One scoop of the Juice+Four Meal Replacement Formula is often recommended to be mixed with the fresh juice of four medium carrots and two medium apples. It makes a great tasting drink, but rather than simply using this recommendation, experiment and find some other juices you like. Here are a few to get you started:

Sunshine Cocktail

2 apples
4-6 strawberries

Lemonade

4 apples
¼ lemon, with skin

Waldorf

1 stalk celery
2 apples

Liver Mover

2 or 3 carrots
½ beet

Digestive Special

handful spinach
6 carrots

AAA Juice

6 carrots
1 apple
2 stalks celery
½ handful wheat grass
½ handful parlsey
½ beet

Cantaloupe Shake

1 cantaloupe, with rind, cut into strips

Alkaline Special

¼ head cabbage, green or red

Potassium Broth

1 handful spinach
1 handful parsley
2 stalks celery
4-6 carrots

Bromelain Special

1 pineapple, cut into strips (with rind, remove top)

Love Apple Cocktail

3 large firm tomatoes
½ cucumber
1 stalk celery
1 small slice lime, with peel

Evening Regulator

2 apples
1 pear

Body Cleanser

4 carrots
½ cucumber
1 beet

Passion Cocktail

4 strawberries
1 large slice pineapple
1 bunch black grapes

The Fresh Juice Advantage

Juicing fresh fruits and vegetables with your own juice extractor provides numerous nutritional advantages that are extremely important to weight loss. Especially during weight loss, the body needs a rich supply of protein, carbohydrates, essential fatty acids, vitamins and minerals. Fresh juice, the liquid extracted from fruits and vegetables, provides this concentrated nutrition which is easily absorbed. If the body is not fed, it feels that it is starving. The result: metabolism will slow down and less fat will be burned. Juicing is an excellent way to supply key nutrients to the body. You cannot get the same effects from canned, bottled, boxed or frozen juices, which have lost most of their nutritional benefits in processing. The juice must be fresh.

The Importance of Raw Foods

Diets containing a high percentage of uncooked foods are significantly associated with weight loss, improved blood sugar control, and the lowering of blood pressure.[26,27] Researchers seeking to determine why raw food diets produce these effects have concluded:

> *A raw food diet is much more satisfying to the appetite.* Cooking can cause the loss of up to 97 percent of the water-soluble

vitamins (B vitamins and vitamin C) and up to 40 percent of the fat-soluble vitamins (A,D,E and K). Since uncooked foods, such as juices, contain more vitamins and other nutrients, they are more satisfying to the body. The result is reduced calorie intake and weight loss.

A raw food diet has a lowering effect on blood pressure. While the blood pressure lowering effect of raw foods is most likely due to their fiber and potassium content, the effect of cooking the food cannot be ruled out. When patients are switched from a raw food diet to a cooked diet (without changing the content of calories or sodium) blood pressure rapidly increases to pre-study values.

A diet composed of an average of 60 percent of the calories ingested from raw foods reduces the body's stress in digestion and absorption of food. Specifically, the presence of enzymes in raw foods, the reduced allergenicity of raw foods, and the effects of raw foods on our gut-bacteria ecosystem are thought to be much more healthful than the effects of cooked foods.

Equally important to good health are the anutrients—food compounds which are not sources of energy themselves, but are of immense value to the body. These are enzymes; pigments like carotenes, chlorophyll and flavonoids; and numerous other accessory food components. Juicing fresh fruits and vegetables is the best way to supply your body with these valuable food components. Enzymes are protein molecules that are responsible for speeding up chemical reactions. Enzymes are what make us alive and are what gives plants life. Plant pigments, especially carotenes and flavonoids, are remarkable in their ability to protect our cells from damage. Fresh juice also contains many other accessory food components which can help fight cancer and promote health.

Juicing fresh fruits and vegetables does provide some fiber, particularly the "soluble" fiber. Although fiber is important, fiber refers to indigestible material found in plants; it is their juice that nourishes us. Our body actually converts the food we eat into juice so that it can be absorbed. Juicing helps the body's digestive process and allows for quick absorption of high quality nutrition. The result? Increased energy levels. This is one of the great advantages of the Juice+Four Super-Nutrient Weight-Loss Plan. Unlike other diets that leave you feeling tired and lifeless, the Juice+Four Plan will provide you with sufficient energy. Energy you can use to burn more calories with physical activity.

You cannot get this energizing effect from canned, bottled, boxed or frozen juices. These juices have been pasteurized, a process which gives them longer shelf life, but causes the loss of identifiable nutrients like vitamins and minerals, as well as the loss of other factors not yet fully understood. Fresh juice is far superior to these juices. Fresh juice not only contains greater nutritional values, it contains enzymes and other biologically active factors.

Whole Foods vs. Processed Foods

In order to achieve and maintain weight loss, foods in their whole or natural form must be a major part of the diet. Highly processed junk foods must be eliminated. The orange is a good illustration of the wide spectrum of foods and food products available, from fresh whole foods to highly processed refined food products, offered in the American food supply.

At each step in this modern evolution of the orange, nutritional value is lost. For example, the vitamin C content of pasteurized orange juice is extremely unreliable. Like most processed juices, their total nutritional quality is substantially lower than that of fresh juice. This is particularly true for juices stored in paperboard containers lined with wax or polyethylene. These products will lose up to 75 percent of their vitamin C content within three weeks.[1] Frozen juice concentrates fare no better and orange drinks have no vitamin C unless it is added. This highlights the fact that in the latter stages listed above, not only is nutritional value lower, there is an increasing number of synthetic additives. More and more food addi-

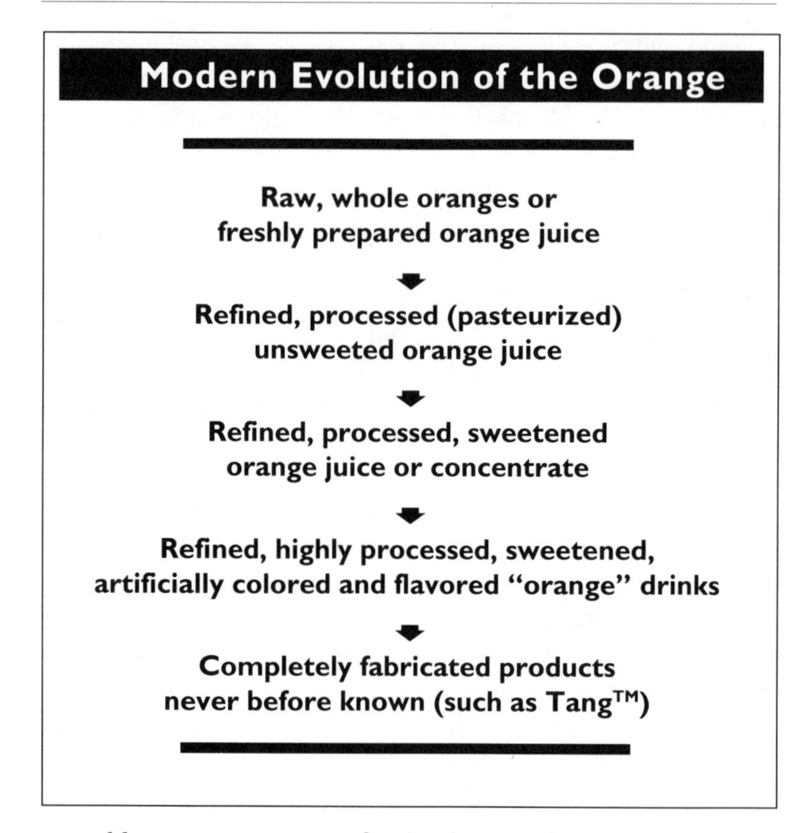

tives, like preservatives, artificial colors, artificial flavorings and acidifiers, are being shown to be extremely detrimental to health. Although many food additives have been banned because they have been shown to be cancer causing compounds, a great number of regularly used synthetic food additives are being linked to such diseases as depression, asthma, allergies, hyperactivity and learning disabilities in children, and migraine headaches.

Maintaining Nutritional Value

Like processing, home handling and cooking also means a loss of the nutrients that are so important during weight loss. For example, upon cooking, leafy vegetables will lose up to 87 percent of their vitamin C content, while carrots, potatoes and other root vegetables will lose up to 33 percent of their vitamin B_1, 45 percent for B_2, 61 percent for B_3, and 76 percent of their vitamin C.[28] However, food doesn't have to be cooked to lose its nutritional value. Food will also lose nutritional value if exposed to air. For example, if you slice a cantaloupe and leave the slices uncovered in the refrigerator, they will lose 35 percent of their vitamin C content in 24 hours.[28] Freshly sliced cucumbers, if left standing, will lose between 41 and 49 percent of their vitamin C content within the first three hours.[28] From this information, we can conclude that it is best to drink juice as soon as it is prepared. However, if this is not possible, fresh juice should be stored in an air-tight container in the refrigerator or in a thermos.

Some juices are better than others for promoting weight loss. The most beneficial juices are those that are dense in nutrients, but low in calories. Here in descending order are the most nutrient-dense fruits and vegetables suitable for juicing:

1. Bell peppers
2. Parsley
3. Kale
4. Broccoli
5. Spinach
6. Celery
7. Brussels sprouts
8. Cauliflower
9. Carrots
10. Cabbage
11. Beets
12. Pineapple
13. Cantaloupe
14. Watermelon
15. Tomatoes
16. Apples
17. Strawberries
18. Pears
19. Oranges
20. Grapes

The first eight vegetables listed are not only dense in nutrients, they are quite powerful. Mixing them with carrot or tomato juice will make them much more palatable. Notice that the fruits are further down on the scale than the vegetables. Although fruits are full of valuable nutrients, they contain more natural sugars than the vegetables and should be juiced less frequently.

The New Four Food Groups

Unlike most diets, the Juice+Four Super-Nutrient Weight-Loss Plan allows a great deal of freedom and flexibility in choosing what foods to eat and when to eat them. The healthy diet component of this system stresses the New Four Food Groups (vegetables, fruits, grains and legumes). These foods contain valuable nutrients and dietary fiber compounds that have important weight-loss promoting properties. The solid meal guidelines that follow, in addition to two daily Juice+Four meals, provide adequate but not excessive quantities of protein.

Avoidance of food components detrimental to health, such as sugar, saturated fats, cholesterol, salt, food additives, alcohol and agricultural residues like pesticides and herbicides, is strongly recommended. The healthy foods recommended are divided into the following categories:

- Vegetables
- Fruits
- Breads, Cereals and Starchy Vegetables
- Legumes
- Additional Protein Sources
- Fats
- Sweeteners

Vegetables

Vegetables are fantastic "diet" foods as they are very high in nutritional value, but low in calories. Vegetables are excellent sources of vitamins, minerals and health-promoting fiber compounds. The following vegetables may be eaten in their raw state, as juice, in salads or steamed. The vegetables noted with an asterisk (*) are termed "free foods" and can be eaten in any desired amount because the calories they contain are offset by the number of calories your body burns when digesting them. In addition, these free foods help to keep you feeling satisfied between meals.

In addition to the vegetables being consumed as juice in a Juice+Four meal, you should eat (or juice) at least four cups of vegetables daily, with one of these cups being a dark leafy vegetable. Additional amounts can be eaten if they are chosen from those marked by an asterisk. Buy vegetables that are in season and eat a variety of vegetables for nutrient diversity. Starchy vegetables like potatoes are included in the "Breads, Cereals and Starchy Vegetables" category.

Vegetable	Calories per cup
*Alfalfa sprouts	20
Artichokes, steamed heart and leaves	44
Asparagus, 6 med. spears	21
Beets	54
*Bell peppers	22
*Bok choy	20
Broccoli	40
Brussels sprouts	54
*Cabbage, green or red:	
raw	24
cooked	31
Carrots	46
*Celery	17
*Cauliflower	27
Chard	30
*Cucumber	16
Daikon radish	26
Eggplant, cooked	38
*Endive	10
*Escarole	10
Garlic, per clove	10
Greens:	
beet	36
collard	40
mustard	40
turnip	29
Jicama	49
Kale	37

Vegetable	Calories per cup
Kohlrabi	40
Leeks	53
*Lettuce	10
*Mushrooms	20
Okra, per 8 pods	36
Onions	50-60
Parsley	26
Peas	106
*Radishes	20
Rhubarb	50
*Spinach	41
*Sprouted mung beans	21
String beans, green or yellow	31
Summer squash (yellow)	40
Tomatoes	23
*Turnips	36
Watercress	7
Zucchini	25

Fruits

Fruits make excellent snacks as they contain fructose or fruit sugar. This sugar is absorbed slowly into the bloodstream which allows the body more time to utilize it, so it is less likely to be stored as fat. Fruits are also excellent sources of vitamins and minerals, as well as health promoting fiber compounds. However, fruits are typically higher in calories than vegetables, so their intake should be restricted somewhat on a weight-loss plan. In addition to the fruit consumed with Juice+Four, one of the following servings of fruit can be eaten during the day or utilized in juice form:

Apples	1 large or 2 small
Applesauce, unsweetened	1 cup
Apricots, fresh*	4 medium
Apricots, dried*	8 halves
Bananas	1 small
Berries:	

blackberries	1 cup
blueberries	1 cup
cranberries	1 cup
raspberries	1 cup
strawberries	3 cup
Cherries	10 large
Dates	4
Figs, fresh	2
Figs, dried	2
Grapefruit	1
Grapes	20
Mangos	1 small
Melons:	
cantaloupe	½ small
honeydew	¼ medium
watermelon	2 cups
Nectarines	2 small
Oranges	2 small
Papayas	1 small
Peaches	2 medium
Persimmons, native	2 medium
Pineapple	1 cup
Plums	4 medium
Prunes	4 medium
Raisins	4 tbsp
Tangerines	2 medium

Breads, Cereals and Starchy Vegetables

Breads, cereals and starchy vegetables are classified as complex carbohydrates. Chemically, complex carbohydrates are made up of long chains of simple carbohydrates or sugars. This means the body has to digest or breakdown the large sugar chains into simple sugars. Therefore, the sugar from complex carbohydrates enters the bloodstream more slowly, so blood sugar levels and appetite are better controlled.

Unrefined complex carbohydrate foods, like breads and cereals made from whole grains and starchy vegetables, are higher in fiber and nutrients but lower in calories than foods high in simple sugars, like cakes and candies. One of the following servings of a complex carbohydrate can be eaten per day:

Breads (from whole grains whenever possible):

bagel, small	1
dinner roll	2
english muffin, small	1
tortilla, 6 inch	2
whole wheat bread	2 slices
rye bread	2 slices
pumpernickel bread	2 slices

Cereals (from whole grains whenever possible):

bran flakes	1 cup
cornmeal, dry	4 tbsp
cereal, cooked	1 cup
flour	5 tbsp
grits, cooked	1 cup
pasta, cooked	1 cup
puffed cereal, unsweetened	2 cup
rice or barley, cooked	1 cup
wheat germ	½ cup
other unsweetened cereal	1½ cup

Crackers (from whole grains whenever possible):

arrowroot	6
graham , 2½" square	4
matzo, 4" x 6"	1
rye wafers, 2" x 3½"	6
saltines	12

Starchy vegetables:

corn	⅔ cup
corn on cob	2 small
parsnips	2 cups
potato, mashed	1 cup
potato, white	1 medium
squash: winter, acorn or butternut	1 cup
yam or sweet potato	½ cup

Legumes

Legumes are fantastic weight-loss foods. They are rich in important nutrients for proper metabolism. Legumes help improve liver function as shown by their cholesterol-lowering actions. Legumes have also been demonstrated to be effective in improving blood sugar control. Since obesity has been linked to loss of blood sugar control (insulin insensitivity), legumes appear to be extremely important in a weight-loss plan. These are some of the key reasons the Juice+Four Meal Replacement Formula provides protein from legume sources.

One cup of the following cooked beans can be eaten each day:

Black-eyed peas	Chick peas
Garbanzo beans	Kidney beans
Lentils	Lima beans
Pinto beans	Split peas
Tofu	Other dried beans and peas

Animal Products

To prevent breakdown of muscle during weight loss, protein intake must be adequate. Juice+Four, along with the plant foods recommended above, will provide more than enough protein. Although we stress the New Four Food Groups, we realize it is necessary to give you some guidelines if you choose to eat some animal protein, especially during the transition phase of improving your diet for better health. Certainly, you should limit animal protein to no more than two servings per week. In addition, if you choose one of the following foods, it will be necessary to reduce your fat selection to one-half serving, reduce by half your breads, cereals and starchy vegetables selection, and eliminate your legume selection for that day.

Fish:

cod	6 oz
sole	6 oz

halibut . . . . 6 oz
salmon . . . . 6 oz
tuna, packed in water . . . . 6 oz
red snapper . . . . 6 oz
perch . . . . 6 oz

Beef (lean cuts):
veal . . . . 4 oz
chipped beef . . . . 4 oz
chuck steak (flank, plate) . . . . 4 oz
tenderloin . . . . 4 oz
plate ribs, round (bottom, top) . . . . 4 oz
rump, all cuts . . . . 4 oz
spare ribs . . . . 4 oz
tripe . . . . 4 oz

Lamb (lean cuts):
leg . . . . 4 oz
rib . . . . 4 oz
sirloin . . . . 4 oz
loin (roast and chops) . . . . 4 oz
shank . . . . 4 oz
shoulder . . . . 4 oz

Poultry (without skin):
chicken . . . . 4 oz
turkey . . . . 4 oz

Dairy:
nonfat milk . . . . 2 cups
2% milk . . . . 1 cup
low-fat yogurt . . . . 1 cup
cottage cheese, low fat . . . . ½ cup

Fats

Fat intake should be reduced to a minimum since fats are very dense in calories. If you can do without extra fat, this is best. One of the following may be consumed each day:

Avocado, 4" diameter . . . . ⅛

Vegetable oil:
canola . . . . 1 tsp
olive . . . . 1 tsp

corn	1 tsp
safflower	1 tsp
soy	1 tsp
sunflower	1 tsp
Olives	5 small
Almonds	10 whole
Pecans	2 large
Peanuts:	
spanish	20 whole
virginia	10 whole
Walnuts	6 small
Butter	1 tsp
Salad dressings	2 tsp
Mayonnaise	1 tsp

Sweeteners

Sweeteners should also be restricted. Again, if you can do with out sweeteners, this is best. One of the following can be eaten each day:

Honey	1 tbsp
Jams, jellies, preserves	1 tbsp
Maple syrup	1 tbsp
Molasses	1 tbsp

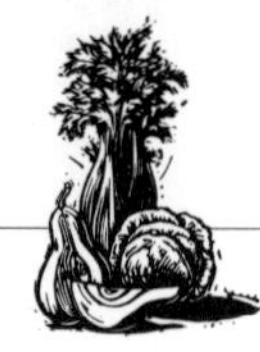

Conclusion

Permanent, healthy weight loss is possible with the Juice+Four Super-Nutrient Weight-Loss Plan because this comprehensive system addresses the underlying factors contributing to obesity. The plan focuses on giving the body the quality of nutrition it truly desires rather than depriving it. The central feature of the plan is fresh fruit and vegetable juice made with your home juice extractor, fortified with the Juice+Four Super-Nutrient Meal Replacement Formula. These, along with the other components of the plan—psychological support, physical exercise and healthy food choices from the New Four Food Groups—work together in helping you create an optimum diet and lifestyle for effective weight loss and weight maintenance.

Remember, by supplying your body with better quality nutrition, the quantity of calories your body needs will be reduced. With improved quality of nutrition, you will improve the quality of not only your health, but your life.

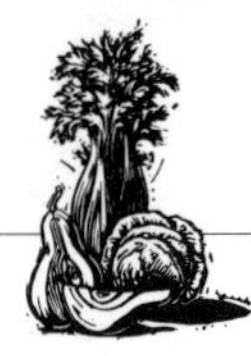

References

1 Shils ME and Young VR: *Modern Nutrition in Health and Disease, 7th Edition.* Lea and Febiger, Philadelphia, PA, 1988.

2 Bray GA: Obesity: definition, diagnosis and disadvantages. *Med J Australia* 142:52-8, 1985.

3 Bjorntorp P: Classification of obese patients and complications related to the distribution of surplus fat. *Am J Clin Nutr* 45:1120-5, 1987.

4 Ashwell M, Cole TJ and Dixon AK: Obesity: new insight into the anthropometric classification of fat distribution shown by computed tomography. *Br Med J* 290:1692-4, 1985.

5 Gillum RF: The association of body fat distribution with hypertension, hypertensive heart disease, coronary heart disease, diabetes and cardiovascular risk factors in men and women aged 18-79 years. *J Chron Dis* 40:421-8, 1987.

6 Contaldo F, di Biase G, Panico S, et al: Body fat distribution and cardiovascular risk in middle-aged people in southern Italy. *Atherosclerosis* 61:169-72, 1986

7 Williams PT, Fortmann SP, Terry RB, et al: Associations of dietary fat, regional adiposity, and blood pressure in men. *JAMA* 257:3251-6, 1987.

8 Haffner SM, Stern MP, Hazuda HP, et al: Role of obesity and fat distribution

in non-insulin-dependent diabetes mellitus in Mexican Americans and non-Hispanic whites. *Diabetes Care* 9:153-61, 1986.

9 Dietz WH and Gortmaker SL: Do we fatten our children at the television set? *Pediatrics* 75:807-12, 1985.

10 Raymond CA: Biology, culture, dietary changes conspire to increase incidence of obesity. *JAMA* 256:2157-8, 1986.

11 Foreyt JP, Mitchell RE, Garner DT, et al: Behavioral treatment of obesity: results and limitations. *Behavioral Therapy* 13:153-61, 1982.

12 Kolata G: Why do people get fat? *Science* 227:1327-8, 1985.

13 Bennett W and Gurin J: *The Dieter's Dilemma.* Basic Books, New York, NY, 1982.

14 Trowell H, Burkitt D and Heaton K: *Dietary Fiber, Fiber-depleted Foods and Disease.* Academic Press, New York, NY, 1985.

15 Thompson JK, Jarvie GJ, Lahey BB and Cureton KJ: Exercise and obesity: etiology, physiology, and intervention. *Psychol Bul* 91:55-79, 1982.

16 Pollack ML, Wilmore JH and Fox SM: *Exercise in Health and Disease.* WB Saunders, Philadelphia, PA, 1984.

17 American College of Sports Medicine: Position statement on proper and improper weight loss programs. *Med Sci Sports and Exerc* 15:ix-xiii, 1983.

18 Oscai LB and Holloszy JO: Effects of weight changes produced by exercise, food restriction or overeating on body composition. *J Clin Invest* 48:2124-8, 1969.

19 Lennon D, Nagle F, Stratman F, et al: Diet and exercise training effects on resting metabolic rate. *Int J Obes* 9:39-47, 1988.

20 American College of Sports Medicine. *Guidelines for Graded Exercise Testing and Prescription, 3rd Ed.* Lea and Febiger, Philadelphia, PA, 1986.

21 Hill JO, Schlundt DG, Sbrocco T, et al: Evaluation of an alternating-calorie diet with and without exercise in the treatment of obesity. *Am J Clin Nutr* 50:238-54, 1989.

22 Farmer ME, Locke BZ, Mosciki EK, et al: Physical activity and depressive symptomatology: the NHANES 1 epidemiologic follow-up study. *Am J Epidemiol* 1328:1340-51, 1988.

23 Gwinup G, Chelvam R and Steinberg T: Thickness of subcutaneous fat and activity of underlying muscles. *Am Int Med* 74:408-11, 1971.

24 Wilmore JH: Alterations in strength, body composition and athropometric measurements consequent to a 10-week weight training program. *Med Sci Sports* 6:133-8, 1974.

25 Ballor DL, Katch VL, Becque MD and Marks CR: Resistance weight training during calorie restriction enhances lean body weight maintenance. *Am J*

Clin Nutr 47:19-25, 1988.

26 Douglass JM, Rasgon IM, Fleiss PM, et al: Effects of a raw food diet on hypertension and obesity. *South Med J* 78:841-4, 1985.

27 Douglass JM and Rasgon I: Diet and diabetes. *Lancet* ii:1306, 1976.

28 White PL and Selvey N: Nutritional Qualities of Fresh Fruits and Vegetables. Futura Publishing, Mount Kisco, NY 1974.

29 Energy and Protein Requirements. A report of a Joint FAO/WHO/UNU Expert Consultation. Technical Report Series 724. World Health Organization, Geneva, Switzerland, 1985.

30 Sarwar G, Savoie L, Peace RW: 'A comparison of in vitro enzymatic and rat balance methods for measuring digestibility of protein and amino acids in foods.' In: Friedman M, ed: *Absorption and Utilization of Amino Acids in Foods.* CRC Press, Boca Raton, FL, 1989.

31 Young VR: Soy protein in relation to human protein and amino acid nutrition. *J Am Diet Assoc* 91:828-35, 1991.

32 Scrimshaw NS, Wayler AH, Murray E, et al: Nitrogen balance response in young men given one of two isolated soy proteins or milk proteins. J Nutr 113:2492-7, 1983.

33 Verrillo A, de Teresa A, Giarusso PC, et al: Soybean protein diets in the management of type II hyperlipoproteinaemia. *Atherosclerosis* 54:321-31, 1985.

34 Sharmanov TSH, Kadyrova RKH and Salkhanov BA: The use of a soy protein isolate in the diet therapy of patients with alimentary obesity. *Vopr Pitan* 2:27-9, 1990.

35 Van Raaij JMA, Katan MB, West CE, and Hautvast JGAl: Influence of diets containing casein, soy protein isolate, and soy concentrate on serum cholesterol and lipoproteins in middle-aged volunteers. *Am J Clin Nutr* 35:925-34, 1982.

36 Carrol KK: Review of clinical studies on cholesterol-lowering response to soy protein. *J Am Dietetic Assoc* 91:820-7, 1991.

37 Redgrave TG: Dietary proteins and atherosclerosis. *Atherosclerosis* 52:349-51, 1984.

38 Beynen AC, Van der Meer R and West CE: Mechanism of casein-induced hypercholesterolemia: primary and secondary features. *Atherosclerosis* 60:291-3, 1986

39 Anderson JW and Bryant CA: Dietary fiber: diabetes and obesity. *Am J Gastroenterol* 81:898-906, 1986.

40 Rossner S, Zweigbergk DV, Ohlin A and Ryttig K: Weight reduction with dietary fibre supplements. Results of two double-blind studies. *Acta Med Scand* 222:83-8, 1987.

41 Shearer RS: Effect of bulk producing tablets on hunger intensity and dieting pattern. *Curr Ther Res* 19:433-41, 1976.

42 Hylander B and Rossner S: Effects of dietary fiber intake before meals on weight loss and hunger in a weight-reducing club. *Acta Med Scand* 213:217-20, 1983.

43 Simonoff M: Chromium deficiency and cardiovascular risk. *Cardiovascular Research* 18:591-6, 1984.

44 Anderson RA, Polansky MM, Bryden NA and Canary JJ: Supplemental-chromium effects on glucose, insulin, glucagon, and urinary chromium losses in subjects consuming controlled low-chromium diets. *Am J Clin Nutr* 54:909-16, 1991.

45 Cooper J, Anderson BF, Buckley PD and Blackwell LF: Structure and biological activity of nitrogen and oxygen coordinated nicotinic acid complexes of chromium. *Inorganica Chemica Acta* 91:1-9, 1984.

Trillium Nutrition Series

These new Trillium Nutrition Series books, by Michael T. Murray, N.D., give you the latest nutrition information, plus recommendations for reducing your risk of diet-related diseases and achieving optimum health.

The Juice Advantage emphasizes the same statement that the Surgeon General, the Sectretary of Health and Human Services, the National Cancer Institute and many others are also making: *"Eat more fresh fruits and vegetables!"* Fruits and vegetables contain proteins, carbohydrates, vitamins, minerals and other key nutrients that are vital to the health of your body. Dr. Murray explains why juicing is such a simple and effective way to add their nutritional advantages to your diet. *#1038. $9.95.*

Eating For Health explains how vital our diet is in determining our level of health and in preventing a wide range of diseases and common health complaints. Dr. Murray answers the important question: "What is a healthy diet?" and provides the very latest scientific information on diet, nutrition and health. Here's everything you need to know to make good food choices for a healthier, happier life. *#1039. $9.95.*

Eating for Arthritis Relief explores the current research linking diet to the treatment and prevention of osteoarthritis, rheumatoid arthritis and gout. While current medical drug treatments often merely suppress the symptoms of arthritis, Dr. Murray explains how using natural measures can address the underlying causes of arthritis for real relief. An explanation of the causes, symptoms and therapeutic considerations for these forms of arthritis is followed by practical dietary recommendations that have proven beneficial in prevention and treatment. *#1045. $9.95.*

A Meal in a Glass!

Juice+Four Super-Nutrient Meal Replacement

Juice+Four blends easily with your favorite fresh fruit or vegetable juices to make a nutritionally complete, low calorie, low fat, high fiber meal—in seconds! This pure, concentrated, easy-to-absorb, vegetarian "super-food" was created in accordance with the New Four Food Groups for healthy weight loss, increased vitality and simple, convenient nutrition.

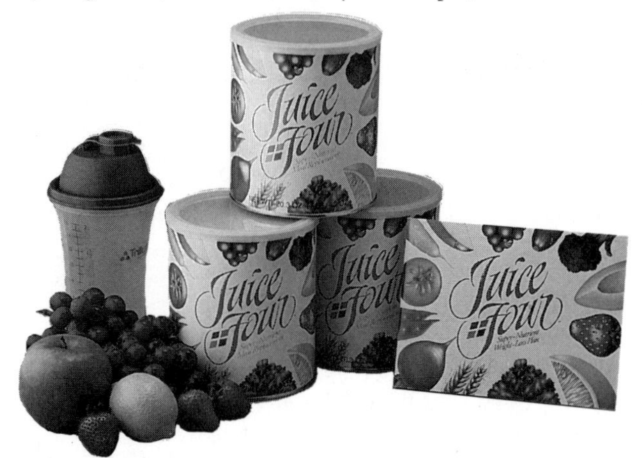

Juice+Four provides a nutrient-packed, healthy balance of. . .

All the essentials:
- Vitamins
- Minerals
- Complex carbohydrates
- Essential fatty acids
- Soluble and insoluble fiber
- Blend of plant-based proteins

With none of the detractors:
- No animal or dairy products
- No cholesterol
- No harmful additives
- No added sugars or flavors—so it won't mask the delicious taste of your juice!

This complete Juice+Four package includes a 3-can pack of Juice+Four Super-Nutrient Meal Replacement (21 servings each), the *Juice+Four Super-Nutrient Weight-Loss Plan* booklet, and a handy 16-ounce Juice Shaker (with an ingenious spoked insert to evenly distribute dry ingredients).

Complete package. #2220. **$89.95** *(a $98.85 value; save $8.90).*

For fast phone orders, call 1-800-800-8455.
Or write: Trillium Health Products, 655 South Orcas, Seattle, WA 98108.